Alkaline Diet: The 21st Century Guide To Alkaline Diet Recipes and How To Maximize The Alkaline Diet Benefits!

Disclaimer

The Publisher has strived to be as accurate and complete as possible in the creation of this report, notwithstanding the fact that she does not warrant or represent at any time that the contents within are accurate due to the rapidly changing nature of the Internet.

While all attempts have been made to verify information provided in this publication, the Publisher assumes no responsibility for errors, omissions, or contrary interpretation of the subject matter herein. Any perceived slights of specific persons, peoples, or organizations are unintentional.

In practical advice books, like anything else in life, there are no guarantees of income made. Readers are cautioned to rely on their own judgment about their individual circumstances to act accordingly.

This book is not intended for use as a source of legal, business, accounting or financial advice. All readers are advised to seek services of competent professionals in legal, business, accounting and finance fields.

Table of Contents

Introduction

About Dieting Based On Alkaline Foods

Normally when people think of dieting on alkaline foods, they consider eating foods without any care of the pH level. The truth would be that these principles could be totally different. Provided you are looking to eating only foods that will balance body pH level, there may be a few steps you ought to take in an attempt to accomplish your objectives.

I hope to analyze the journey to dieting on alkaline foods effectively. However, I could strengthen you for a unique level of victory. Please consider several thoughts one ought to anticipate before looking to alkalize the body with alkaline foods. Yes, before dieting on alkaline foods, you ought to gauge and verify that alkalizing the body is the right direction for you.

Now, the easiest method to make that assessment would be to ask yourself the following questions:
Do you have the ability to follow through on a diet plan?

Do you stick to a plan no matter whatever to see it through? - *Do you have a determined personality that will not be distracted from set goals?*

Hopefully, your answer to the questions was "yes". Those habits are typical among folks who are into alkaline diet foods. You have already taken the first big step towards dieting on alkaline foods!

Nevertheless, note that dieting on alkaline foods will not likely be the hardest part of the diet program. In fact, dieting on alkaline foods would be a lengthy process which takes around 5 days to prepare. It would be sensible to be as equipped as possible before getting started.

However, here are some instructions to push you to begin:

Making Sure You Are Aware Of the Acid Forming Foods

Making sure you are aware of the acid forming foods is so vital because without doing this, you could get wavering. That could result in becoming unable to achieve alkaline diet foods impact. There are a few traits that individuals ought to have in an attempt to alkalize the body with alkaline foods. So folks with these traits should already make sure you are not ignorant of the acid forming food either regularly.

Studying Various Alkaline Forming Foods

Studying various alkaline forming foods helps you achieve alkaline diet better. Understandably, it could be tough to get in the habit of doing this. But you can start by studying various alkaline forming foods a day, and this should become habitual when you are on alkaline diet foods.

Stuffing Your Pantry With Alkaline Forming Foods Will Be A Good Place To Start...

The key to doing well with dieting on alkaline foods would be reliant upon stuffing your pantry with alkaline forming foods. This will be a good place to start..., yet many individuals do not interpret just how important this really is! Though stuffing your pantry with alkaline forming foods will be a good place to start.... by doing that you make certain that you're equipped with alkaline diet foods.

Without doubt, dieting on alkaline foods takes somewhat more than waking up one evening to say, "Hey, I need to diet on alkaline forming foods." Perhaps that is a start. However, to gain any success with dieting on alkaline foods, you should initially invest mentally.

Dieting On Alkaline Foods - A Look Back

If you have thought about dieting on alkaline foods, you definitely have a tough road ahead. If it was simple, everyone would achieve it. Most individuals who decide to alkalize their body with alkaline foods end up not actually seeing it through.

Don't think of eating foods without any care of the pH level. The truth is that, dieting on alkaline foods needs an individual to be perseverant and strong-willed. We know this. Now we are able to review the stages recommended with dieting on alkaline foods so we could appreciate our upcoming success.

You should probably take this day to check whether you have the ambition it requires to really do this. Do you have a perseverant attitude? It would be an important part of the process that everyone who expects to diet on alkaline foods need, otherwise alkalizing the body could be extremely tough, if not beyond reach.

You have previously also examined if you are tenacious once you were asked: Do you stick to a plan no matter whatever to see it through? I congratulate you on making it to this distance, because this means you apparently have not given up. This is a major difference between doing one thing and hoping to do it. That will come up frequently in alkalizing the body.

You asked those targeted questions and looked deep within your spirit to determine if you possess exactly what is necessary to diet on alkaline foods. And you have done a good deal to prepare.

You see, most individuals who have failed dieting on alkaline foods did so because all of them were not totally equipped. But, through seeing if you have what it takes to diet on alkaline foods ahead of time, you have invested your spirit in moving along.

The reason for this is that dieting on alkaline foods requires your mental stamina just as much as it requires your physical stamina. Clearly, dieting on alkaline foods would be extremely physical, but just by maintaining a stable mind you could prepare yourself for success.

For as many decades as dieting on alkaline foods has been around, the people who have done so successfully had one obvious thing in common. They appreciated precisely what was necessary, and were surely ready to tackle it head on.

What may we learn from this? Well, if you are equipped to diet on alkaline foods, I mean, once you prepare, you'll be capable of overcoming this challenge, and nothing could stop you!

Without a doubt, it is a fact that not all people are informed about the health benefits of alkaline diet to the body. The truth is that people just eat foods that they like with little or no understanding of its implications to their health.

Now, there is no gainsaying that living healthy begins from the food that we eat. Well, a major thing you may have to consider as you journey in life is to live a life free from illnesses by applying yourself to a healthy diet regime. Several individuals have benefited from their diet plan and one of the most powerful ways is to follow a good alkaline diet plan.

As you will find out, this is a type of diet plan that has cured some people who have illnesses like arthritis, Cyst, and those who suffered from obesity and weakness.

Generally speaking, sickness is regarded as a hindrance to our everyday lifestyle of living. But, the truth is that, if an individual is sick, he or she is just not able to accomplish much, if anything at all!

And as a matter of fact, sickness may commence from living an unhealthy lifestyle as a result of what you eat.

Now, let's face it, in order for our body to function well, the pH balance should be maintained and then the regular pH of the body fluid must be steady at 7.3.

Well, that can be achieved by maintaining an alkaline condition of the body fluid and not allowing the body to develop total acidic fluid which is usually harmful to the body system.

Moreover, to balance the body alkaline pH state seamlessly, the first and foremost thing to do is to acquire the knowledge of alkaline forming foods and get used to them, as the basis for your type of meals choice.

The truth is that by having the right knowledge of this list of foods, it would be very feasible for you to always come up with the right alkaline recipe that will work for your body.

Without any doubt, I want to say that increasing the consumption of alkaline foods is a proven strategy that have helped a great deal in curbing the unabated surge in the amount of acids inside our body. Now, by consuming alkaline foods, I mean the foods that are rich in alkaline pH.

The import of the above is more obvious as we know that the acidic-alkaline balance is a must for the body to be healthy and to maintain it in a healthy working condition that will consequently lead to a stress free life. To achieve that balance, expert recommends the 80-20 ratio. That is, the consumption of 80% alkaline foods and 20% acidic foods.

Now, in case the pH balance of the body is tilted towards the acidic side, then the body becomes susceptible to numerous sorts of ailments ruining the nervous system.

But, if you have been harboring the desire to alkalize your body and you are running out of ideas, then the following are numerous ways that you can resort to get to your goal.

First and foremost, to alkalize the body, the very first step needed is to have adequate knowledge of list of diet foods that are rich in alkaline. Then, you need to know how these foods and their alkaline contents affect the body to rightly apply them.

Then, considering the fact that vegan's diet, which are more of fruits and vegetables, are rich in alkaline, you will need to consume a lot of them.

However, you need to be careful, because there are other fruits and vegetables that are considered to be acidic in nature. This more or less explains why you need to acquaint yourself with the alkaline food list.

The fact is that, if you have the right knowledge of alkaline foods, as you are getting by your reading of this book, you will be confident you are doing the proper thing that will bring positive changes to your life.

And by applying the alkaline diet program, you will be assured that you are consuming stuffs that will bring a fantastic effect to your body wellness.

The Alkaline Diet plan

Searching to find the advantages of starting by using an alkaline diet plan? A lot of people include created stories to the truth that they are gaining huge health advantages coming from these kinds of diet plans, between elevated vitality to fat reduction to osteoarthritis alleviation or even trying to keep hassles and in some cases cysts away.

Plan Meals Ahead

Really, presently there seem to be a huge amount of folks around obtaining advantages from trying to keep their particular human body's pH on or even close to high level. Hence the dilemma can be, just what do you have to complete and keep ones alkalinity at bay?

Furthermore, you'll find that over time, you'll get faster and more comfortable at knowing what you can and can't eat. Something that often helps is writing a list of your meals at the beginning of the week by sitting down for an hour with a list of foods or recipes. From there, you can just follow the list so you won't have to constantly be thinking when you're hungry.

Young people can often get away with abusing their bodies, but older bodies are not as resilient. One area of concern is that will kidney functionality typically decline together with age?

For the reason that kidneys have the effect of excreting the excess acidity manufactured by any low-alkaline diet plan, and lessened kidney functionality can cause one's body to become additional acidic. In turn, a build-up of acidity in the body can put seniors at increased risk of various health problems.

One of these health problems is osteoporosis, which is at least partly caused when the body withdraws alkaline minerals from the bones in order to mop up excess acid.

This process, which might sound self-destructive, helps to keep acid from building up too much, but at the price of bone loss. The best way to cope with this problem is to follow an alkaline diet, which prevents the acid from being formed in the first place.

Eat Your Fruits and Veggies

The foods that are most commonly high in alkalinity are certain fruits and vegetables. Some of my favorite high-alkaline fruits include apples, oranges, blackberries, watermelon, and bananas. For vegetables, I tend to rely heavily on carrots, celery, baked potatoes, mushrooms, and eggplant.

Once you're on the diet, you can begin including some more variety into it, but the important thing is to get started quickly and easily. Over time, tweaking your diet will bring you to a fully rewarding alkaline lifestyle.

Remember the Importance of Balance in Alkaline Diet Plan

A good rule of thumb would be going 75% alkaline foods and 25% foods with low acidity; in fact, we can apply the 80-20 principle here without any doubt and you will be fine. Well, the truth is that you're almost never going to want to eat the highly acidic foods, but to be honest; an occasional treat is not a huge problem.

The bottom line is that it's about balance, just like anything else. Some people are quite successful by planning a diet where on 6 days of the week they eat a strict alkaline diet plan, and on the 7th day they will treat themselves to some of the acidic "no-no" foods so that they feel a reward for all the healthy eating that they accomplished throughout the week.

Alkaline Diet Energy - Its Curing Power

Alkaline diet is a diet, which is fundamental in reaction and is generated by the mix of alkaline salts, including sodium bicarbonate. Robert O. Young promoted this diet as part of releasing his book "The pH Miracle".

Its roots lie in microbiology, sports science, plant-based nutrition and longevity studies.

The Characteristics of Alkaline Diet

Alkaline diet is replete with vegetables, alkalizing water, fruits and lean meats such as salmon. It involves a holistic approach to enhancing overall health through consuming foods with an alkali content that mimics the human body's customary pH level of 7.36 to 7.44.The normal alkaline diet energy should be a mix of 80% alkali and 20% acidic.

The ideal way of implementing alkaline diet is to have breakfast of an alkalizing meal.

How Good Is Alkaline Diet Energy?

People who have changed their diets from the traditional diet to the alkaline diet have witnessed thunderous benefits such as happiness, energy, respite from joint pain and overall health. In fact, alkaline diet energy is conducive for those who wake up in the morning with fatigue.

A strict adherence to alkaline diet energy lowers the risk of several health issues like heart failure, stroke, cardiovascular disease and cancer. Besides, it has the capacity to lessen symptoms of poor health, such as hives and weak nails and excess mucus generation. It halts the aging process of individuals. More importantly, alkaline foods yield positive results as they cut down acid levels in the body.

Why Alkaline Diet Energy Is Recommended For Use?

The idea behind consuming diet rich-aided alkalizing foods is to restore balance to the body. Besides, it inhibits recurrent colds and infections.

It brings down circulating levels of acidic compounds in the body by recommending a minimal intake of foodstuffs that have abundant levels of acid, for example meat and enhancing the intake of items with low levels of acid, such as potatoes and mushrooms.

Eating an alkaline diet alters the blood pH minimally and transiently. On top of this, alkaline diet energy aids in avoiding processed foods, white flour, white sugar and caffeine.

Alkaline Diet Energy Chart

Vegetables: A diet proficient in vegetables is one form of simplest ways to quickly reinstate the body's pH balance. Green vegetables such as spinach, broccoli, kale, green beans and arugula are among the most effective alkalizing food items.

Traditionally, alkaline diet energy has supported measures like avoiding meat, cheese, poultry and grains so as to make urine more alkaline(higher pH), altering the environment of the urine to stop kidney stones and persistent urinary tract infections.

Fruits: Avocados, grapes, lemons and water melon are the four essential fruits that contain alkaline diet.

Also, available health evidence says that a diet with less acid-producing foods like bread and animal protein help a lot in checkmating cancer besides strengthening bones.

Adverse Effects

On the other side, alkaline diet energy causes certain ill effects too. Since the alkaline diet energy promotes certain categories of food, there is a potential danger of resulting in having a complete balanced diet which might cause nutrient deficiencies such as phytonutrients and vital fatty acids.

Can the Alkaline Diet Prevent Cancer?

The Alkaline Diet is one of the latest diet crazes sweeping the world. It seems like new diet fads have been introduced to the public on a non-stop basis for years now. Have we finally found the one that can help us fight cancer, cholesterol, and just poor health in general?

You should know that there are many positive things about the alkaline diet. It encourages the intake of more fruits and vegetables, which is shown to have health benefits in any diet.

Also, if you are at all familiar with alkaline food charts, you will see that the "safe" foods are not processed or high-starch foods. Studies have found that processed foods may at least be influential in the development of cancer.

However, the base of the alkaline diet, which claims that eating highly acidic foods raises the pH levels of your blood, are not accurate. The first place that food goes to be digested is your stomach, which contains some of the most powerful acid known to man.

From there, the food enters a process in which components end up either in your excretory system or your circulatory system. Within this process, your body works hard to keep the pH level of your blood balanced. The acidity of your urine can change, but the pH in your blood will maintain balanced levels.

This doesn't mean that the diet will not help you to be healthier and even possibly prevent cancer. The medical community doesn't know where cancer starts or originates, though it is certain that some are genetically predisposed to it.

However, professionals believe that a healthy diet and exercise routine can help to delay the onset of cancer at the very least. The foods that are recommended in the alkaline diet are mainly composed of uncooked vegetables and some fruits. Many vegetables lose some of their nutritional value when cooked, so eating them raw proves a healthier option.

Similarly, the alkaline diet recommends avoiding things like processed sugar, processed grains, and processed foods in general. Well, there have been multiple studies done into processed foods and their effect on your body, and the findings in all of these studies was that processed foods are not a healthy option.

In fact, at the very least, they have been shown to increase fat content and bad cholesterol in our body. And at most they may be responsible for things such as heart problems, high cholesterol, and even cancer.

There is also a possibility that a steady diet of highly acidic foods increase the chance of kidney stones. While this is not cancer, it's also not something that you would find pleasant if you ever have to pass through such an experience.

So, whether or not the philosophy behind the alkaline diet is correct, there are demonstrable health benefits to sustaining diet. These health benefits are certain to include lower risk of high blood pressure and high cholesterol, and may include reduced risk of cancer. If you are looking for a viable option for a healthy diet plan to follow, the alkaline diet is a good place to start.

Alkaline Diets for Vegans

With the constant advocacy for people to turn and lead healthy eating lifestyles, people are now readily reducing on indulgence of overly fatty or processed food stuffs. Some people nonetheless take this a step further and actually embrace a vegan lifestyle.

As a common knowledge, going vegan for an individual requires a lot of dedication to completely avoid and eliminated the eating of all dairy, meat and poultry products and choosing to only eat vegetables, fruits and grain foodstuffs.

However, in the recent past, some dieticians have come up with a new level of vegan lifestyle of adopting and only eating an alkaline diet for vegans.

So What Exactly Consists Of An Alkaline Diet?
The concept behind the alkaline diet is based on pH optimization balance. By avoiding certain food products and drinks like caffeine, artificial and processed foods one gets to eliminate rotting and fermenting foods from the system.

The perception is that, it is a superior diet and thus enables an individual live a vibrant lifestyle eliminating common complaining conditions like poor sight, memory loss, weight gain and creaking of bones especially in old age.

In the alkaline diet, eliminating all kinds of food stuffs including bread, cheese, mushrooms, vinegar and soy sauce is recommended. It is presumed that it is kinder on the overall digestive system as the food stuffs are of the same pH as the blood stream.

Benefits Attributed With the Embracing Of an Alkaline Diet for Vegans

Persons who have embraced this kind of lifestyle have expressed various benefits which they attribute to the alkaline diet. They include

•Reduction of coronary diseases infections

•*Reduction and alleviation of diabetics' condition and symptoms*

•Fast recovery in the event of previous stroke attack

•*Loss of weight and maintenance of proper weight. This has been attributed to the higher number of anti-oxidant rich fruits and vegetables that enable individuals maintain a relatively ideal BMI thus leading to overall smaller waist line.*

•Increase in lean muscles and maintenance of the same which leads to increase in metabolism of an individual

•*Reduction in injury as individuals have expressed confidence that they have grown stronger*

•Finally it has enabled many people achieve a younger appearance. This is due to reduction and elimination of processed sugar that reflects in lower blood sugar levels thus leading to increased skin elasticity

Concerns That Arose Regarding the Alkaline Diet

Because of the numerous restrictions on what one can and cannot eat, various dieticians have raised concerns of how healthy and practical the alkaline diet is. However, due to limited research the claims below are still merely a speculation

   •*Concerns of the quantity of calcium and vitamin D: This is a great concern as the diet eliminates various sources that were thought to be ideal*

   •The alkaline diet has been flagged as unsuitable especially for pregnant women given the fact that they don't get the needed vitamins and minerals needed to support a healthy pregnancy

   •*Foods that are rich in iron that help in blood cells formation like bread, pulses and certain grains is eliminated*

   •With Vitamin B12 mostly gotten from animal sources, taking of supplements to ensure a healthy blood, and nervous system is recommended.

Alkaline Diet Recipes

In the recent years alkalinity has emerged as one of the natural ways to stay fit. It helps you lose weight and stay away from various diseases. The alkaline diet mainly consists of food items that contain calcium, iron, manganese, zinc and copper.

Have you ever sat down and thought how the ancient people rarely experienced many diseases like we do and how healthy they were? Specialists who deal with alkaline diet issues have done research on the difference between the ancient food and the modern food diet and have come up with startling results.

They help get rid of aches and pains, poor digestion, diseases and low energy as well. Increasing your consumption of salads and fresh vegetable juice is a good way to control the acidic environment in your body. If you get a few of these signs you need to start alkalizing your body.

A lot of ancient food consisted of alkaline diet recipes that would balance the acidic with the alkaline. The invention of machines is what brought about processed foods which were acidic.

An acidic diet mainly leads to critical diseases like cancer and diabetes. Research has also been carried out to support this claim. Evidence also shows that cancer cells survive well in an acidic environment. People who have consumed an alkaline diet talk a lot about its effects towards having a healthy body. In fact the alkaline diet has been proposed by a lot of physicians.

In addition, an alkaline diet also consists mostly of citrus fruits, vegetables, nuts, legumes and tubers. The key to getting the right alkaline diet is not eating acidic foods. For you to have the right diet you need to keep away from things like sugar, processed foods starch, caffeine and alcohol.

The moment you start sticking to the diet you will notice great improvement in how you feel, many people say they have more energy and also a smoother skin.

Lack of a diet is not the only thing that causes over-acidification in your body. There are also environmental toxins, recreational drugs, cigarettes and prescription drugs. All these cause acidity in the tissues and blood. Lack of sleep, chronic stress and even negative thoughts can lead to acid in our bodies.

Many doctors agree that people should make use of a diet plan. It isn't rockets science really, just good common sense eating and good alkaline diet recipes supplementation.

The diet is very easy to follow since it goes back to the ancient times when people consumed only natural foods, unlike today where almost everything is chemically made to ensure it is easily preserved.

Therefore an alkaline diet does not involve any recipes to adhere to. All the foods are available in the grocery stores and the only difficult thing will be to forego all the foods you had been accustomed to.

Wrap Up

Now, in conclusion I want you to review the *12 easy ways to remove acid build-up from your body, alkalize your pH and beat disease;* this is an extract from (NaturalNews) http://www.naturalnews.com/... *written by: JB Bardot*

Most of us over the age of five were brought up to believe life is very complicated and our bodies are a jumble of parts, each with a different name and a corresponding ailment; dozens of diets to overcome the effects of highly complex micro-crap called food; and television punctuated with an entire industry of false promises and dark demons hawking medicines for lesions we didn't even know we had.

The end result of this twisted perspective is an outlook that dissects humans, infuses each and every cell and fiber with acidosis and creates disease as the result of a lack of wisdom and the truth.

As a result of our misguided beliefs, most of us are walking cells of battery acid in leaky vials waiting to overturn or to turn over into the grave.

Humans were never meant to be carved up into miniscule parts, each to be treated as separate from one another. Each molecule, cell and organ is meant to communicate with each other; and yes, the foot bone really does connect to the brain bone.

The holistic bodily system that pulls us all together and keeps us healthy and functioning optimally is not a system at all, or even a concept... it's our blood pH. When the pH is balanced, the body is healthy.

Most disease states can't exist when the body's pH is alkaline. Bacteria, viruses and fungi can't reproduce. So what's a body full of fast foods, drugs, GMOs, and non-organic food to do?

Get alkaline and balance your pH

1. Choose only organic foods that are GMO-free to avoid pesticides, chemicals and other contaminants

2. Eat alkaline foods like most fruits and vegetables. They sustain the body's pH on a daily basis.

3. Reduce all kinds of meats, fowl and refined sugars and flours. Protein intake should be approximately 40-50 grams daily. These foods contribute to an acidic state.

4. Combine highly alkaline foods in a meal with foods that are acidic to create better balance and maintain alkaline pH.

5. Drink one or two glasses of organic apple, cider, vinegar and water daily. Mix one to two tablespoons of vinegar in eight ounces of water.

6. Make a pH drink by combining two tablespoons lemon or lime juice with half a teaspoon of baking soda. After foaming has subsided, add 8-12 ounces of water and drink immediately.

7. Add one to two teaspoons of baking soda mixed with an eight ounce glass of water daily. If you have hypertension or edema, this may not be a good choice for you. Speak to your health practitioner.

8. Consume foods high in potassium like lemons, bananas and honey.

9. Lemonade or lemon water helps to clear the body of excess acids and create an alkaline-forming state. Mix the juice of half an organic lemon with two teaspoons of raw honey and eight ounces of warm water. Drink first thing in the morning to flush the system. Do not warm water in microwave oven.

10. Mix one to two teaspoons cream of tartar with eight ounces of water. Cream of tartar is very acidic, like lemons, and helps to create an alkaline-forming state. It is especially good to use in an emergency, to quell nausea, relieve a headache or overcome shock. It has a light, sour taste and is very refreshing mixed with room temperature water. Do not sweeten.

11. Drink lots of water daily to flush the system of waste. Consume in ounces, 50 percent of your weight in water every day. In other words, if you weigh 150 pounds, drink 75 ounces of water daily.

12. Supplement with digestive enzymes to help balance the body's pH and overcome acidosis. The pancreas is responsible for producing most digestive enzymes, including bicarbonate. If your pancreas is not functioning properly, the quantities of natural enzymes can be less than optimal.